How to Eat Your Best Life

Tawnee Saunders

I dedicate this book to my kids and grandkids for enduring my endless nutrition discussions and insights over experimented-on and continually morphing food concoctions. This book is also dedicated to my family for loving me just the way I am. Also, I want to thank my friends and clients who ask for more and believe in me.

Contents

Introduction

This book is a reflection of my health, fitness, and life journey and the excitement I have about sharing it with the world. It is my hope and desire you will find in these insights and recipes who you are and what you are capable of. Remember, all that life really takes is *practice*. I believe in each one of you with all of my heart. I want this to be the beginning of wherever you are going next.

The recipes you will find in these pages are very liberal. This is 100% intentional! That is because they are more than recipes. They are exercises in empowerment!

It is critical to your mindset to see these recipes as "exercises" in making the affirmations to which they are attached. The purpose of these exercises is to give you choices, but also to help you practice thinking outside the box.

Through these affirmations and food exercises, I bring you insight and experience from my work as a life, nutrition, supplement, and fitness coach. I'm also a mother, grandmother, friend, podcaster, and positivity pusher. My daily goal is to spread positive inspiration everywhere: from social media to my personal life.

I want to support you, all those around me, and everyone in the world to live their best life.

How to Use this Book

1. Treat this book like a mini master class. Find a comfortable place to read. Block out distractions. Think about the messages.

- What things resonate with you? Which do not?
- What is your own story? Is it anything like mine?
- How do you feel about what you are reading?
- Are you panicking over the freedom I'm giving you in the recipe? Are you stuck in your old food ways?

2. After every chapter and exercise, I want you to **record what happened, what you felt, and what you learned!** There's room in the book to annotate, but you can also get a companion journal for the book by visiting http://www.tawneesaunders.com/printables. Or, just go buy a journal of your own!

3. Make notes! Bring your colored pencil and your sticky notes. The things you are about to read are going to bring inspiration and memories to your mind. You are going to want to write them down.

4. This is a learning opportunity! Remember, freedom, creativity, empowerment, and learning are the goal. So, embrace your personal power and creativity. Your choices may, or may not, give you your desired results. Learn from every practice, and make a plan to try again.

5. Involve friends. Choose a chapter and affirmation. Do it for breakfast, lunch, or dinner. Send out invites to friends. Print off journal pages to share also! (see http://www.tawneesaunders.com/printables).

- Welcome everyone to the party with a healthy beverage.
- Divvy out meal preparation tasks to the group as you begin to prepare the meal.
- Have at least one person (or more) read through the chapter you choose to focus on.
- Have a discussion about the reading. Share insights and inspiration. Journal together.
- Eat a fun, group-created meal.

6. Give the book as a gift! I'm a fan of a "Just Because" bag. I've been doing it for years. Here is what goes inside of it and how to do it.

- Find a plain gift bag that costs around $1. Make sure it will hold the book and a few additional items.
- Place the book inside along with a variety of goodies and snacks. Choose small bags of nuts, cranberries, or raisins. I love when a goodie bag has a small bottle of water or another healthy beverage inside. Maybe include a travel-size lotion or hand sanitizer. Be creative!
- Cost of book + bag + treats = a wonderful gift between $15-20.
- Print a fun "Just Because" card from http://www.tawneesaunders.com/printables to attach to your bag!

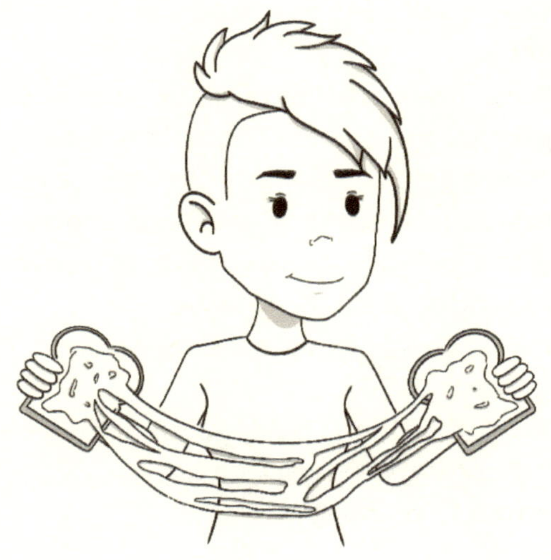

I Am Unique

Record your thoughts!

1. What makes you different from everyone else?
2. How does being different make you feel?
3. Do you think being different, or unique, is ok?
4. Why do you want to be the same as someone else?

____

____

____

____

____

____

I am unique. You are unique.

Over the past several years, I have tried one health-fitness-diet philosophy after another, only to get discouraged when it wouldn't work for me like it did for someone else. So, after a lot of discouraging tries, and many times of hoping for the same results, I realized that despite many similarities, when it comes to health and nutrition none of us are the same.

So, what did I do? I decided that from every presented health theory or diet, I would take away all of the golden nuggets that work for me. The rest I simply leave behind. I stopped expecting the same results that others may have gotten. Now I look instead for my own unique results.

When it comes to food lifestyle, supplements, and really all that life offers, I have stopped comparing myself, my life, and my results to others. We are all on our own timeline. I love that there is just one of me! You need to learn to accept and love that there is just one of you.

As you make this recipe, I want you to say out loud the phrase:

I am unique!

I chose a grilled cheese recipe for I Am Unique because it is a recipe that is easy to make unique for you! Tweak the bread or the cheese. There are so many variations! It's delicious, healthy, simple to make, and brings comfort. You will fall in love with this recipe and your unique self.

I Am Unique – Grilled Cheese Sandwich Exercise
This is an exercise in embracing that you are unique.

Step 1: Choose a bread:

Sourdough, 100% whole wheat, sprouted whole grain, rye, _______________

Step 2: Choose a cheese(s):

Swiss, mozzarella, blue cheese, cheddar (white or yellow), Havarti, pepper jack, _______________

Step 3: Choose extras:

Bell peppers (any color), fresh baby spinach, sliced meat (ham, beef, turkey, or chicken), avocado, _______________

Step 4: Choose a sauce or seasoning:

Pink salt, sea salt, ground black pepper, chipotle, sriracha, spicy mustard, Thai coconut, avocado ranch dressing, lime juice, _______________

I am unique!

Step 5: Create!

1. Preheat an electric griddle to 350 degrees, or heat up a large frying pan to medium-to-medium-high heat.
2. Use grass-fed butter (e.g. Kerigold) and lightly butter the outside of two slices of bread.
3. Place first slice of bread on heated pan or griddle.
4. Apply sauce, then one slice of your chosen cheese. Then, put on all the other ingredients. Place on top another slice of cheese.

5. Put on the other slice of bread.
6. Press down on the sandwich with a large spatula. Then, cover the sandwich for 1 minute with a large pot lid for quicker melting. Flip when the bottom is golden brown. Repeat.
7. When both sides are golden brown (or darker to taste) remove the sandwich. Let cool 2-3 minutes.

I am unique!

Tip 1: Practice taking moderate bites. Chew at least 10-15 times minimum before swallowing, allowing for all of the flavors to be detected and enjoyed. Repeat until sandwich is gone...and please lick any residue from your fingers!

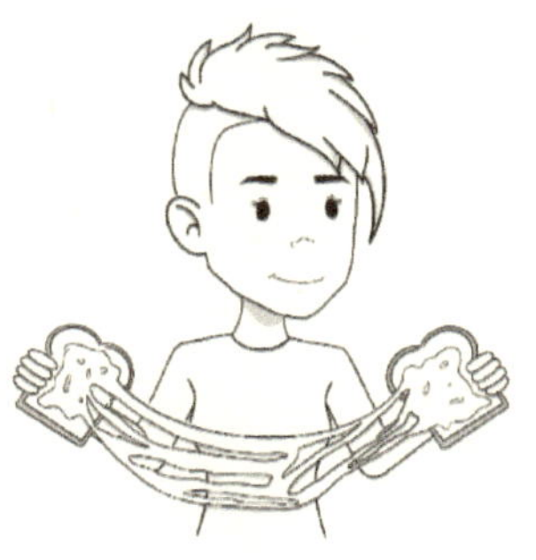

Tip 2: Do no limit yourself to the suggestions above. Use the empty blanks to write in your own ideas. Come up with several crazy and tasty grilled cheese sandwich combinations unique to you!

My Unique Grilled Cheese Variations are:

____

____

____

____

____

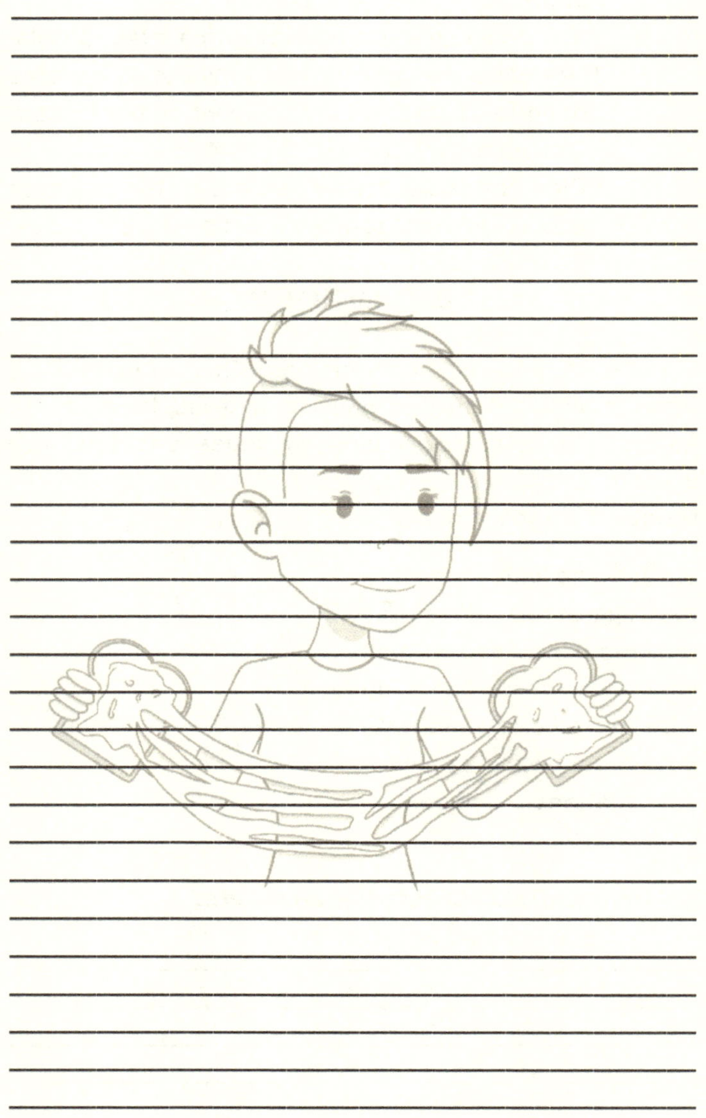

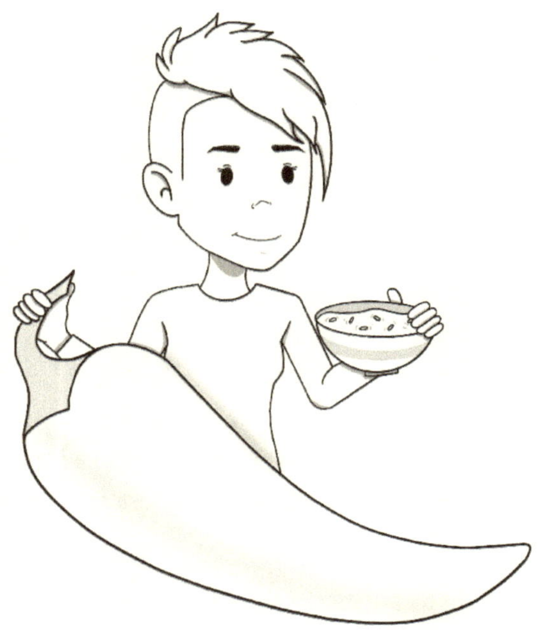

I Am Incomparable

Record your thoughts!

What makes something incomparable? Is it because it is unique? More of something than anything else? Not the same as another?

____

____

____

____

____

Nothing compares to you! You are incomparable. I can't compare my eating style to your eating style.

Most of us spend our whole life comparing ourselves to others. I admit, I did this for countless years. In fact, these are some of the things I said to myself over the years:

- I can't sing like her.
- I can't apply makeup like her.
- Why can't I play basketball like boys?
- Why can't I look as good in that dress as she does?
- Why can't I have the perfect body like that girl?
- Why is my life so hard and others have it so good?

It has taken me many years to realize that I am incomparable to any other person that walks, or has ever walked, this earth. Even though I have learned this, I still find myself hearing that voice in my head from time-to-time. However, now I recognize that voice. I have learned to change those thoughts with firm and positive affirmations like:

- I may not be able to sing like her, but I do have a voice and I'm so grateful for the voice I have.
- I am not a makeup artist. Nor can I draw a good cat-eye. But I look great anytime I do wear my makeup. Wearing makeup or not, I feel great and I'm so grateful for how I look.

I could go on, but you can see where I'm going with this.

Why are firm and positive affirmations so important? Because you are incomparable! There is no other being on this planet that has your mind, body, and soul.

I chose chili for this recipe because there are so many versions of chili out there. There are so many variations, just like we are all human with variations.

As you are creating one of these chili recipes, or crafting your own, I want you to say out loud the phrase:

I am incomparable!

I Am Incomparable – Chili Exercise

I'm going to give you measurement suggestions for various ingredients. But please feel free to experiment! Use your imagination!

Step 1: Choose a meat (preferably grass-fed):

White bean: 1-2 lbs. boneless skinless chicken or ground turkey
Red bean: 1-2 lbs. Beef, bison, or lamb

Step 2: Choose a bean

2-4 cans white, red, or black beans

Step 3: Choose a broth

White bean: 2-4 cups organic bone broth in chicken or vegetable
Red bean: 2-4 cups organic bone broth in beef or vegetable

Start with 2 cups and add more if needed.

Step 4: Choose other ingredients

<u>White bean:</u> two 4 oz. cans chopped green chilies, 1 tsp fresh garlic (or powder), 1 tsp oregano (and/or cumin), 1-3 tbsp. coconut oil/olive oil, cheddar cheese, heavy whipping cream, sour cream, yellow potatoes, chili powder mix (or come up with your own spice mix), salt and pepper to taste, _______________________________.

<u>Red bean:</u> two 4 oz. cans chopped green chilies, a few chopped bell peppers, organic tomato paste (read can/tube for measurement), 1 chopped white or yellow onion, diced tomatoes, chili powder mix, sweet potatoes, _______________________________.

I am incomparable!

Step 5: Create!

1. In a large pot, soften aromatic vegetables (onions, bell peppers) in 1-3 tbsp of your chosen oil. Brown your meat in the same pot after softening your aromatic vegetables.
2. Rinse and drain your beans. Add to pot along with green chilies.
3. Pour in 2-4 cups of bone broth. The more broth you add, the soupier the chili becomes.

Did you know that salt is a flavor amplifier? Without the right level of salt, many spices are hard to taste. Try to get your salt level right before adding <u>unsalted</u> spices. If you use a spice mix, and it has salt, add it first before adjusting the salt level. As well, most broths contain salt. Keep this in mind when adjusting the salt level.

4. Bring to a boil. Add spice mix (or use your own spice mix, or a packet of chili seasoning from the store). Stir 'till combined. Taste the chili for salt and flavor level. If it needs more salt, add ¼ tsp at a time.
5. Simmer for 15-30 minutes.
6. Remove from heat. For white chili add the cream and stir well. Taste for salt and flavor. Adjust as needed.
7. Serve with any type of corn tortilla chips and with an optional garnish of shredded cheese and fresh cilantro.

I am incomparable!

Tip 1: A fun way to eat this, besides a good ol' fork, is with some blue corn chips or any other favorite chip. Scoop it right out of your bowl!

Tip 2: Chili is extremely versatile. Do not limit yourself to the ingredients, spices, and suggestions above. Try to come up with an incomparable version of chili that you create through experimenting!

My Incomparable Chili Recipe is:

____

____

____

____

____

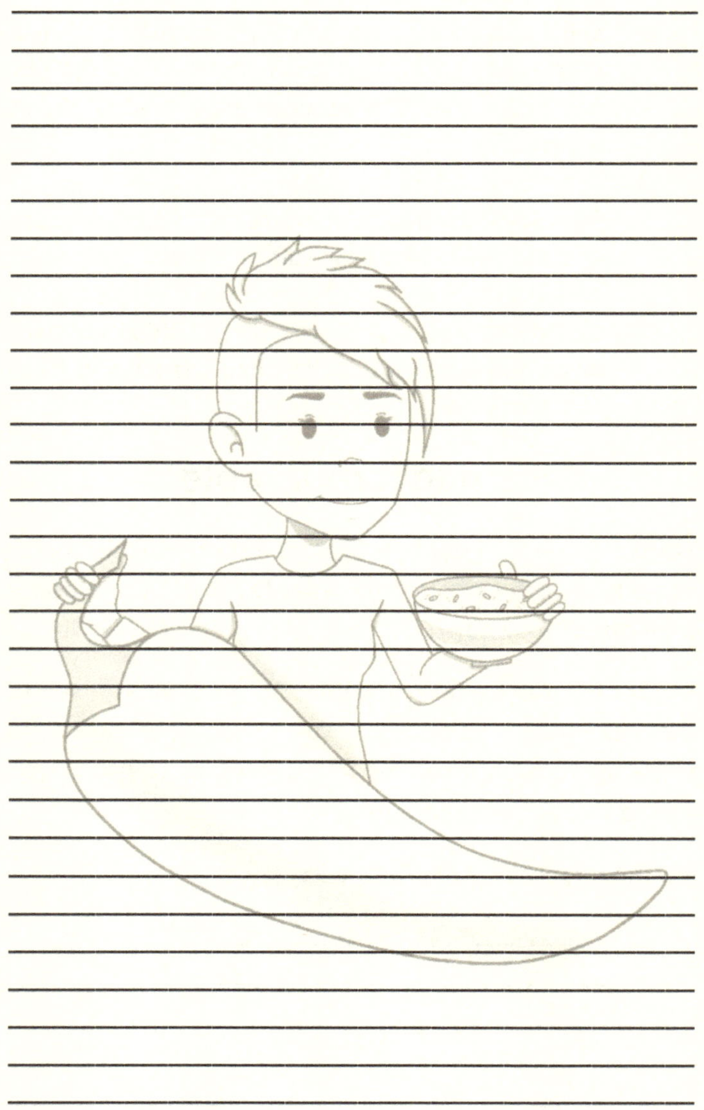

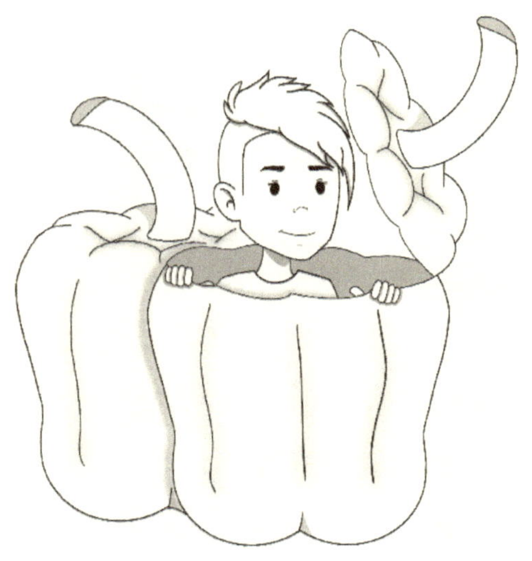

I Trust My Gut

Record your thoughts!

What is my first response to situations or conversations that challenge me? How do I feel? What do I think? Do I trust myself?

____

____

____

____

____

I trust my gut, and so should you!

I have learned that life goes more smoothly when I listen to my body. Everyone is born with an innate wisdom to make decisions and navigate their life.

When I turned 40, my body was always in pain. I thought to myself, "If I feel this way at 40, what is 80 going to feel like?" My body was using pain and discomfort to communicate with me. I knew there were changes I had to make. I knew that if I didn't make those changes my life was going to be tougher than what it already was.

If you learn to tap into your gut thoughts and feelings, you will get a whole new level of wisdom.

I used this opportunity to change. I started to learn, in great detail, about wellness and began to experiment with food and supplements. I began to learn to listen to my body.

For example, bread and pasta are two of my favorite things in the whole world. However, they don't make my body feel good. So, why do I like them? Because I have an emotional connection to them.

Bread is a comfort food for me. Emotionally, it warms me up. It reminds me of the homemade bread my mother made when I was growing up. That was the highlight of my day, when I would come home from school and she would have hot, fresh bread ready for us. Hot homemade rolls at Thanksgiving are a sought-after treat. I love spaghetti because it reminds me emotionally of a birthday dinner with my Grandma way back when I was young. These were the real reasons I ate bread and pasta—not simply curing my hunger.

I chose an Italian Butternut Squash recipe for this gut lesson because, not only is it healthy for my body, but it tastes amazing, and it creates an emotional response of warm feelings for me when I eat it.

My youngest sister introduced me to this recipe. She makes it to warm the soul and delight the senses. She pours love and gratitude into it as she is making it; love of those who will eat it and gratitude for the nutritional goodness is provides, but also gratitude to God for the blessing of being able to have it, make it, and eat it.

As you make and indulge in this mouth-watering recipe, I want you to say out loud the phrase:

I trust my gut!

Why? Because, like me, you too can find healthy, tasty alternatives to foods in your life that don't agree with your gut while also creating warm, cozy memories and feelings.

I Trust My Gut – Italian Butternut Squash Exercise
I'm going to suggest a few possible variations on this recipe. But feel free to experiment!

Ingredients necessary for ALL variations:

- 1-2 cups "Parmesan-Reggiano" cheese, grated. This is an authentic Italian cheese and can be found at Sam's Club, Costco, and in smaller blocks at most grocery stores or delis.

- 1 cup cream (try to find a brand *without* carrageenan added in)
- ½ tsp salt + ¼ tsp black pepper
- 1 Tbsp butter
- 1 bag baby or regular spinach (roughly chopped). You can substitute 1 bag spinach and kale mix (chopped) or ¼ - ½ lb. frozen spinach
- 1 lb. sweet Italian sausage (ground, not links). Johnsonville brand is available at most grocery stores.

Variation 1 – Butternut Squash
<u>Prep time</u>: 30 minutes
<u>Bake/Broil time</u>: 70 minutes
<u>Total time</u>: 1 hour 40 minutes (worth every minute!)

You will need 1 large butternut squash, or 2 small-to-medium butternut squashes. You will also need 2 red bell peppers.

<u>Note</u>: Butternut squash can leave a funny film on your skin. Consider wearing nitrile gloves while slicing.

1. With a good sharp chef's knife, remove the top(s)/head(s) and the bottom(s) of the squash. Cut the butternut(s) in half (approximately) by slicing right above the rounded bottom. Carefully cut off the skin of the squash. If the rounded-bottom flesh is sufficiently thick, consider de-seeding and using, but it is often difficult to use.
2. Cut the large butternut squash in half (longways) and then halve the two halves. You should end up

with four (4) relatively equal pieces. If using two small or medium-size squashes, halve longways but do not halve again.

3. Line a sheet pan with foil. Spray or coat lightly with oil. Spray, or lightly coat, the squash pieces with oil and a sprinkle of salt. Place the squash pieces largest-side down onto the oiled surface.

4. Cover the sheet pan(s) with foil and bake at 400 degrees for 50-60 minutes.

5. While the squash is baking, finely chop the two red bell peppers and throw them in while you brown the ground sweet, Italian sausage. Set aside.

6. Melt 1 Tbsp of butter in a medium saucepan. Add in roughly chopped spinach and wilt. When the spinach is wilted, add 1 cup cream, ½ tsp salt, and ¼ tsp black pepper. Bring to a low simmer (try not to boil the cream). When you see consistent steam rising off the cream, add in the grated Parmesan-Reggiano cheese (1 cup for taste, but add more if you want it thicker and cheesier). Remove from burner and stir until thick and combined. Set aside.

7. When butternut squash is baked (a fork sticks in clean and comes back out without any effort), remove top foil and let cool for about 3 minutes. Gently mash the center of each butternut chunk, but only slightly.

8. Spoon 1-2 Tbsp's of the cheese/spinach sauce onto to each chunk of squash. Then, spoon on 2-3 tablespoons of the Italian sausage mix onto each chunk of squash. Put it back in the oven for 10 minutes under the broiler, on high.

9. Pull out as soon as the sausage starts to brown and crisp. Let cool for 5 minutes before serving. Spoon on additional cheese sauce as desired.

Variation 2 – Sweet Potato
<u>Prep time</u>: 10 minutes
<u>Boil/Broil time</u>: 25-30 minutes
<u>Total time</u>: 40 minutes

You will need 4-8 medium-large sweet potatoes. You will also need 2 red bell peppers.

1. Peel sweet potatoes. Cut in half longways.
2. Boil sweet potatoes 15 minutes or until you can stick a fork in them without breaking them apart.
3. Let the potatoes cool.
4. Finely chop the two red bell peppers and throw them in while you brown the ground sweet, Italian sausage. Set aside.
5. Melt 1 tbsp of butter in a medium sauce pan. Add in roughly chopped spinach and wilt. When the spinach is wilted, add 1 cup cream, ½ tsp salt, and ¼ tsp black pepper. Bring to a low simmer (try not to boil the cream). When you see consistent steam rising off the cream, add in the grated Parmesan-Reggiano cheese (1 cup for taste, but add more if you want it thicker and cheesier). Remove from burner and stir until thick and combined. Set aside.
6. When the sweet potatoes are mostly cool, place them on a foil lined (and lightly oiled) sheet pan. Gently hollow out the middle of each half. Try not to remove the center, but simply make an indentation.

7. Spoon 1-2 Tbsp's of the cheese/spinach sauce into the center of each sweet potato half. Then, spoon on 2-3 Tbsp's of the Italian sausage mix onto each chunk of squash. Put the sheet pan in the oven for 10 minutes under the broiler, on high.

8. Pull out as soon as the sausage starts to brown and crisp. Let cool for 5 minutes before serving. Spoon on additional cheese sauce as desired.

You can also make this version casserole style by slightly mashing the sweet potatoes and putting them in a cake pan and layering the cheese sauce and sausage on top.

I trust my gut!

Variation 3 – Carrots & Potatoes
<u>Prep time</u>: 30 minutes
<u>Boil/Bake/Broil time</u>: 40-45 minutes
<u>Total time</u>: 1 hour 15 minutes

You will need a 1 lb. bag of carrots and/or parsnips, 5-7 yellow (or red) potatoes (no russets) and 1 large sweet yellow onion. This version is a casserole version.

1. Peel carrots and potatoes. Roughly chop carrots and potatoes and boil in salted water for 15-20 minutes. Drain carrots and potatoes and line the bottom of a cake pan. Slightly mash the carrots and potatoes if you want a more even layer.

2. Peel and finely chop the large, sweet yellow onion. Add it in while you brown the ground sweet Italian sausage. Set aside.

3. Melt 1 Tbsp of butter in a medium sauce pan. Add in roughly chopped spinach and wilt. When the

spinach is wilted, add 1 cup cream, ½ tsp salt, and ¼ tsp black pepper. Bring to a low simmer (try not to boil the cream). When you see consistent steam rising off the cream, add in the grated Parmesan-Reggiano cheese (1 cup for taste, but add more if you want it thicker and cheesier). Remove from burner and stir until thick and combined. Set aside.

4. Spoon the cheese/spinach sauce over the top of the carrot/potato layer. Then, spoon on the Italian sausage mix. Spread evenly. Put the casserole pan in the oven and bake for 20-25 minutes.

5. Let cool for 5 minutes before serving. Spoon on additional cheese sauce as desired.

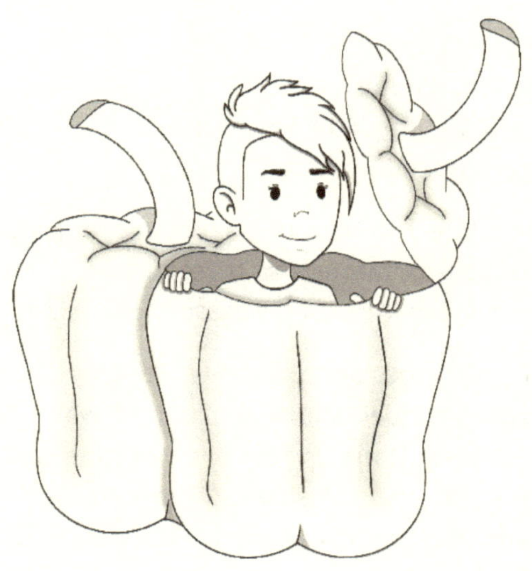

Variation 4 — Stuffed Red Bell Peppers
<u>Prep time</u>: 30-60 minutes
<u>Cook/Broil time</u>: 10-20 minutes
<u>Total time</u>: 1 hour 20 minutes

You will need a red bell pepper for each person. You will also need a large, sweet yellow onion, and cooked white or brown rice.

1. Cook the rice per appliance or package directions. For 4 people you'll need two cups of cooked rice. For more than 4, try for up to 3-4 cups of cooked rice.
2. Cut off the top of the red bell peppers just below the stem. Hallow out the inside, removing all seeds.
3. Peel and finely chop the large, sweet yellow onion. Add it in while you brown the ground sweet, Italian sausage. Set aside.
4. Melt 1 Tbsp of butter in a medium sauce pan. Add in roughly chopped spinach and wilt. When the spinach is wilted, add 1 cup cream, ½ tsp salt, and ¼ tsp black pepper. Bring to a low simmer (try not to boil the cream). When you see consistent steam rising off the cream, add in the grated Parmesan-Reggiano cheese (1 cup for taste, but add more if you want it thicker and cheesier). Remove from burner and stir until thick and combined. Set aside.
5. Fill the peppers 1/3 of the way with cooked rice.
6. Spoon the cheese/spinach sauce over the top of the rice. Be generous. Then, spoon on the Italian sausage mix. Spread evenly. Put the stuffed peppers in the oven and bake at 350 degrees for 20 minutes.
7. Let cool for 5 minutes before serving. Spoon on additional cheese sauce as desired.

I trust my gut!

There has got to be at least 30 more ways this recipe could delight your gut and mine. Play with some substitutions and alternatives and write them down here!

____

____

____

____

____

____

If you love your own version, share it with me on my Facebook Page (Tawnee Saunders)!

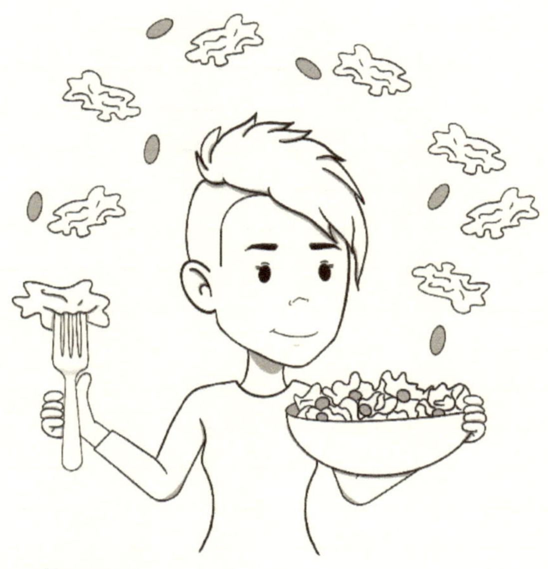

I Have Power

Record your thoughts!

Are you comfortable making a choice? Are you ever afraid to make decisions? Do you often worry about what someone might think of your decisions or choices?

____

____

____

____

____

____

____

I have power. You have power.

We all have power to change our lives. About a year after I really got serious about my health, I had made a significant amount of progress. I had lost 20 lbs. I had energy. My body felt pretty good, certainly much better.

I was driving to work in my car, and I was hungry. I gave into the temptation to stop and get breakfast at McDonalds. I ate it. Every bite I was beating myself up about what was in my mouth and what I was swallowing. I was so mad at myself for my choice. Yet, I kept taking another bite, chewing and swallowing.

I got to work and sat in the car for a few minutes. I was mentally distraught. I looked in the mirror and said out loud, "Why? Why did you do that? What is it going to take to just say no? What is it going to take to be more prepared? What kind of pain do you have to endure before you recruit the power you know you have to make better choices?"

A few tears welled up. I was so frustrated and disappointed with myself. Seriously! All the knowledge I had acquired, all the things I knew about the food I had just put into my body and what it would do to me...why did I struggle with this? I got mad. Looking back on it, I laugh but that is what it took to take me to the next level of commitment.

You have the power within you! Sometimes you just have to find it.

I chose this recipe because there are so many combinations when it comes to salad. Just like there are so many things we go through to learn and grow and find our personal power. It takes personal power to do something different.

So, here's the challenge. Try NOT using lettuce in your salad. Small steps lead to actual habit change.

It takes internal power to do something different. You have the power to make changes.

When you are making this salad, I want you to say out loud:

I have the power to put whatever I want in this salad just like I have the power to make choices in my life.

Make sure your tone is firm and sincere. Say it as many times as you can.

Let me join you in this exercise! Visit http://tawneesaunders.com/videos/

I Have Power— No Lettuce Salad Exercise
Let's be honest, the perfect parts of the salad are not the various kinds of lettuce, even though I enjoy some baby spinach on occasion.

So, what is a salad exactly? A salad is a cold dish of various mixtures of raw, or cooked, vegetables (and fruit) usually seasoned and topped with a dressing made of oil, or oil and vinegar. On occasion, it is accompanied by meat.

With this in mind, I want you to throw out everything you know about salad right now, and let's create something fresh and new!

I have power!

Possible Ingredients (use these or build your own):

- Cucumber
- Shredded carrots
- Roasted chopped sweet potatoes
- Bell peppers (all colors)
- Corn
- Onions (all kinds)
- Black beans
- Lemon juice or lime juice
- Dijon mustard
- Honey
- Olive oil/ coconut oil
- Cayenne pepper
- Cilantro
- Chopped or sliced avocado
- Sliced or chopped tomato
- Berries: strawberries, blueberries, raspberries
- Mandarin oranges
- Salt and pepper to taste
- Seeds: ground flax, chia
- Cheese: all kinds
- Dressings: all kinds

I have power!

Create:

Here's a recipe suggestion to get you started.

In a bowl, combine chopped cucumbers, tomato, cheddar cheese, strawberries, blueberries, avocados, cooked and cooled golden potatoes, chopped bell peppers. Sprinkle lightly with salt, pepper, ground flax and chia seeds. Top with a light mix of coconut oil and your favorite vinaigrette. Pick up a few salad dressings.

Tip 1: Make sure your bowl is filled with amazing colors and flavors.

Tip 2: Do not limit yourself to the suggestions above. Please brainstorm and come up with all kinds of tasty combinations.

My Unique No-Lettuce Salad variation is:

____

____

____

____

____

____

Come up with a great no-lettuce salad? Share it with me on my Facebook page (Tawnee Saunders)!

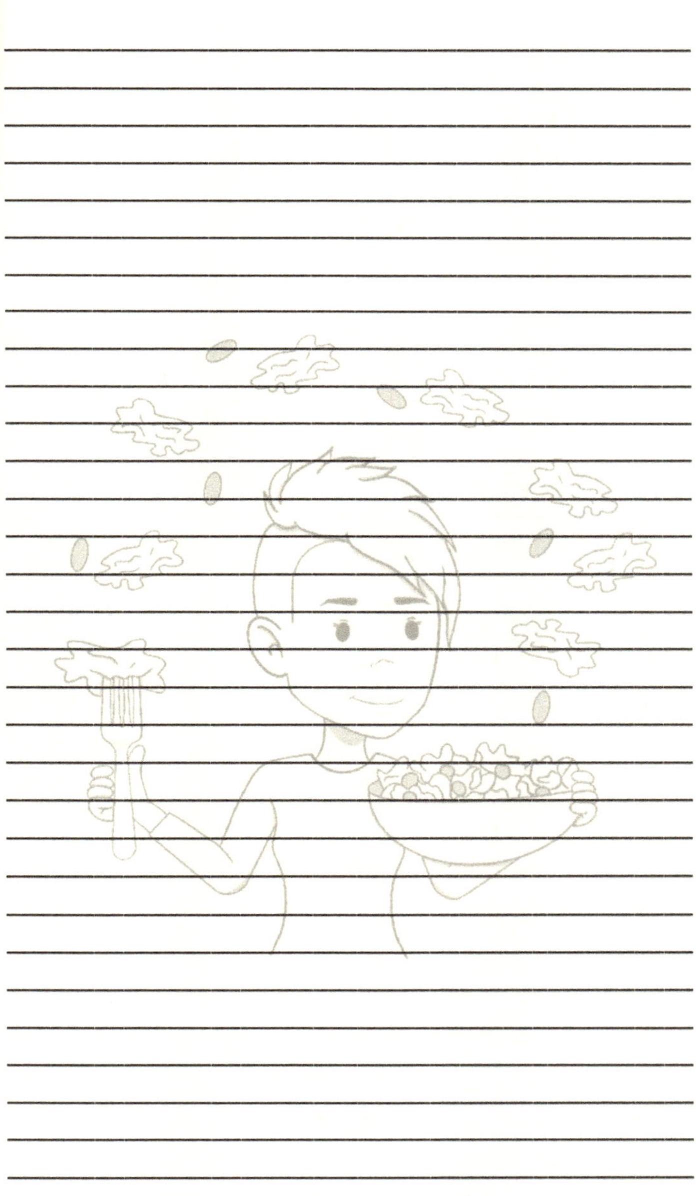

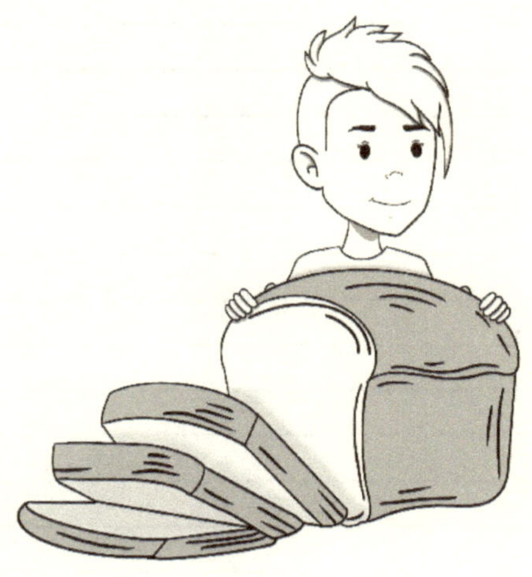

I Am Intuition

Record your thoughts!

Do I listen to my thoughts? Do I ponder my thoughts? Am I creative in my decisions?

____

____

____

____

____

____

We are all intuitive. We know not everything out there is going to work for us. I reject the diet lifestyle. I eat when I'm hungry but I simply make good food choices. I refuse to battle with food. I listen to my body and make intuitive choices. I know when I'm full and I don't force myself to eat extra food.

I allow myself to enjoy food by chewing slowly, enjoying the different textures and tastes, smelling the aroma in the air, and finally swallowing and taking a deep breath. This process brings me satisfaction. When I am happy, I find rewards that don't include food. When I am sad, I also look for comfort in things that don't include food. Through these things I truly respect my body. This also allows me to honor my desire for health and happiness.

This is my intuition. All I have to do is follow it.

I learned this epic lesson in coach training. A whole new world was opened to me. It was all the stuff I already knew intuitively. When we hear the truth, we recognize it. I was so excited to put it into practice.

I remember the first time I sat down to eat. I made sure I didn't have to rush. I actually had to focus on not being in a hurry and counting how many times I chewed each bite of food. It was harder than I expected. I had no idea how mindlessly I went through my day.

I also had a tough time learning how to stop eating when I was full. I grew up learning to clean my plate. As someone who worked hard to put food on the table at my house, every morsel not eaten was wasteful. I had to overcome that as well.

As you make this amazing banana bread, say out loud:

I am intuition!

If you really want to have fun with it, whisper, "I am intuition," as if intuition is whispering in your ear. It takes intuition to make good banana bread as well. Depending on the pan you use, or your altitude (high altitude can affect quick bread recipes significantly) it may need less time to cook, or more time. Adding chocolate chips may change the cook time as well. Watch the bread. Check it with a toothpick. Listen to your intuition.

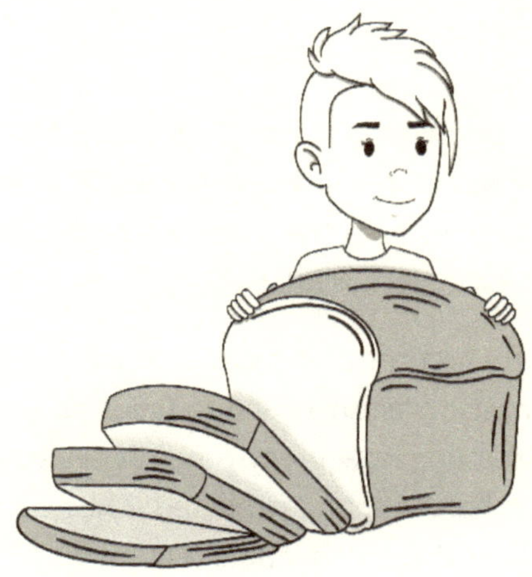

I Am Intuition – Banana Bread Exercise
Ingredients:

- 3 ripe bananas
- ½ cup yogurt (plain or vanilla)
- ½ cup honey
- 1/3 cup coconut oil

- 1 tsp real vanilla (extract is okay too)
- 2 eggs
- 1 ½ cups unbleached white flour, white whole wheat flour, or wheat flour
- 1 tsp baking soda
- 1 tsp baking powder
- ¼ tsp cinnamon (or more to taste)
- ¼ tsp sea salt (because it has more minerals! But regular table salt is fine to get started)
- Optional spices (I always add these):
  - ¼ tsp ground cardamom
  - ¼ tsp ground cloves
  - ¼ tsp ground ginger
  - ¼ tsp ground nutmeg
  - ¼ tsp cumin
- Optional extras:
  - Chopped walnuts, or pecans
  - 1/3 bag of chocolate chips
- Optional nutritional additions:
  - I like to add 3 tbsp of collagen. You can get it in vanilla flavor, but I find buying it in one cannister, non-flavored is best.
  - 1 tbsp ground flax seeds, or chia seeds.

I am intuition!

Create:

1. Preheat oven to 350 degrees.
2. Oil pan(s) with olive oil pan spray. Use pans that heat evenly.
3. Mash bananas (I happen to like to leave mine a little chunky). Add yogurt, honey, vanilla. Mix till

combined. Beat eggs in a separate bowl and mix into wet ingredients until combined.

4. Combine all the dry ingredients. Mix with a whisk to disperse the spices and rising agents well.

5. Combine dry ingredients with the wet ingredients until just combined. Pour into greased pan(s).

6. Bake at 350 degrees for approximately 50-75 minutes (shorter time for shallower cake pans, longer time for deeper bread pans). Keep an eye on it. The time is variable. The outer edges tend to brown and cook faster, but the middle may still be gooey. Use a toothpick to test. Use your intuition. Say...

I am intuition!

7. Once bread is cooked, let it cool for about 30 minutes in the pan. After 30 minutes, use a butter knife to ensure that the bread is not stuck to the sides of the pan. Tip bread out onto a cooling rack or bread board.

This recipe is great warm, drizzled with hot, melted grass-fed butter, or try some melted gooey peanut butter! Honey? Sure! Be creative!

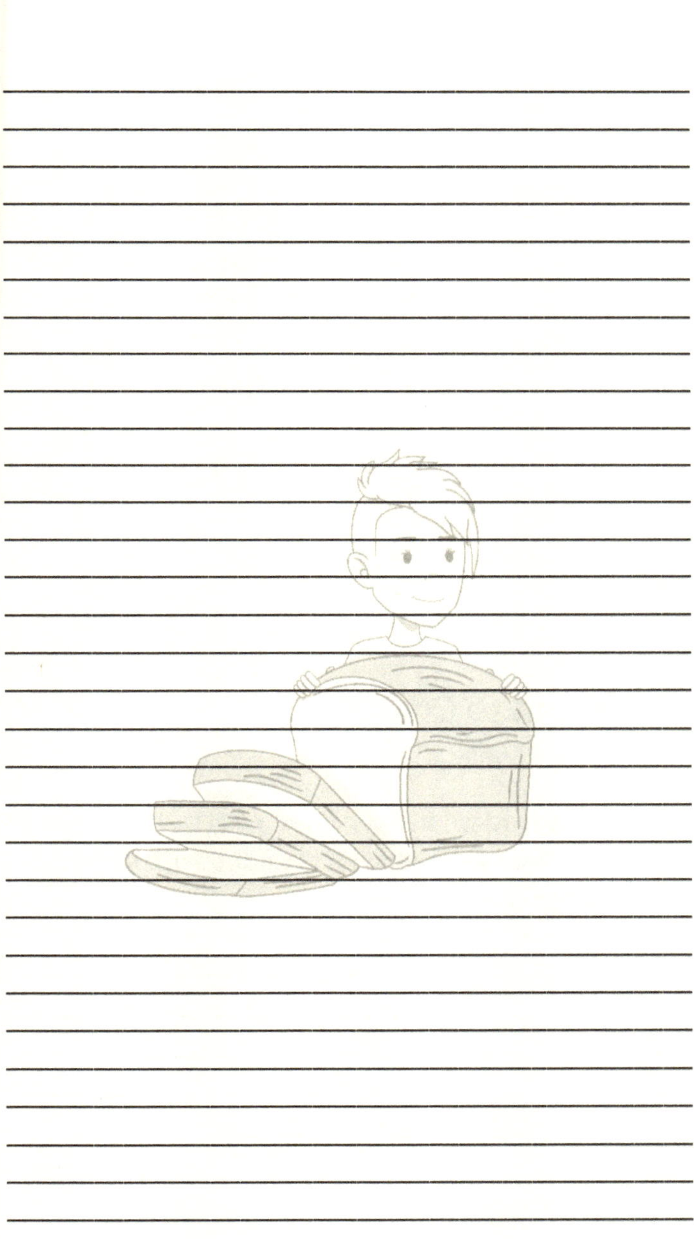

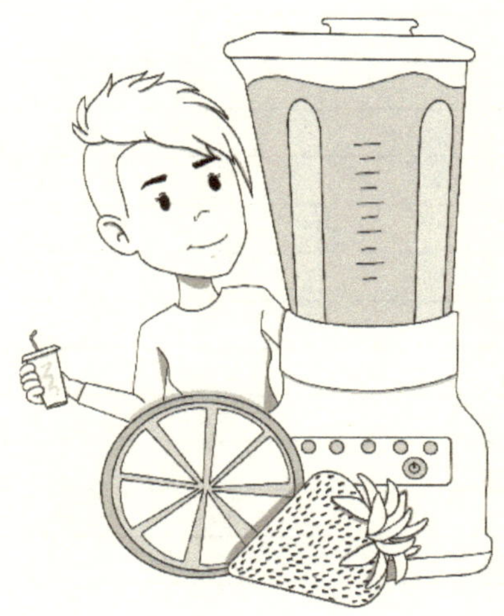

I Am Open to Change

Record your thoughts!

Am I ready for something new? Will I take a chance if I get it? What will happen if I'm not open to a change I know I need?

____

____

____

____

____

I am open to change. You can be open to change.

Most of us think we are open to change until something happens and we realize we have a belief that limits possibilities for us. At the end of 2018, I made the commitment to myself to be open to change. Easily said! I quit a secure job with awesome people because I really wanted to grow. I knew if I didn't jump, I might never get the opportunity to change course.

Within three months I was given the chance to move 1,100 miles away from my family and pursue my dreams. I was so committed to being open to change I didn't hesitate. I packed my SUV till it was bursting and started a new journey. Because I was truly open to change, I now live in an amazing town on the edge of a mountain.

What's funny about this is that I have been saying for years that I was moving to the mountains! But it didn't happen for me until I was truly open to change.

Here, I enjoy counseling clients on life, health, fitness, and nutrition. I get to witness lives change. I have a growing podcast that I get to collaborate with The Doctrine Lady on. We get to meet and interview amazing people whom I would have otherwise never have had the pleasure to meet.

I can say I am living a blessed life that gets better every day. Without being open to change, I would not be able to bring you this fun life-changing book!

I will always be open to change!

As you make this recipe, I want you to say out loud the phrase:

I will always be open to change!

Stand up straight, shoulders back, and say it with intent. Say it as you add each ingredient to this recipe. You will find more confidence and encouragement as you go throughout your day.

Let me join you in this exercise! Visit http://tawneesaunders.com/videos/

I chose smoothies for this bit of encouragement because to craft a fun and healthy smoothie, that you won't ever get tired of, you have to be open to change. Make the suggested recipes, but then make some changes. Try your own! As long as you're open to change there will never be a boring smoothie—ever.

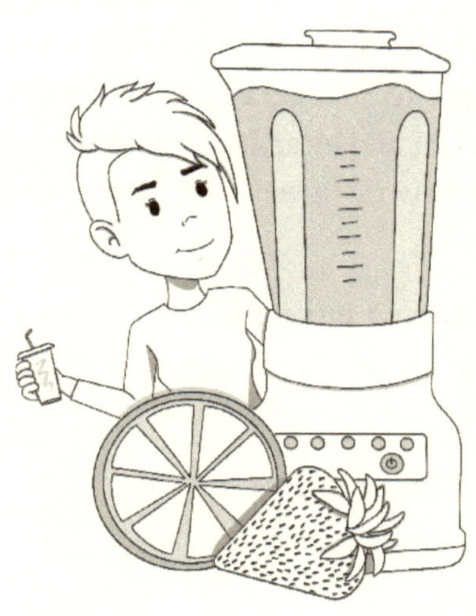

I Am Open to Change – Smoothie Exercise

I'm going to suggest a few possible variations on this recipe. But please experiment! Try to keep out added sugar. It's hard, but you can do it.

Smoothie 1: Chocolate Peanut Butter

Ingredients:

- 1 ½ cups milk of choice (regular or almond)
- 1 tbsp all-natural peanut butter (because it has less sugar), or other all-natural nut butter
- 1 tbsp cocoa powder, organic if possible
- ¼ cup heavy cream (or coconut cream, cashew milk)
- ¼ tsp sea salt (very important to bring out flavors)
- ½ banana, or a handful of dates (this is your sweetener)

Blend, blend, blend.

I am open to change!

Tip 1: Add vanilla protein powder or a few tablespoons of collagen! You can also sneak in ground flax, or chia, seeds. Nuts too! Sky's the limit. If you really want to have some fun, add in some dark chocolate chopped up for some texture. This smoothie should never remain the same.

Tip 2: Try to keep out "added" sugar. The point in these recipes is to make food fun, to take control of the food, but to be more intentional and healthier. With a little thought, most food can still taste amazing and be better for you.

Tip 3: Be brave! Add small amounts of things you normally wouldn't eat but want to put into your day: kale, spinach, or other greens. Make the amounts small to start and work your way up slowly.

Smoothie 2: My "I Am Open to Change" Smoothie

Ingredients:

- 4-8 oz. container of yogurt of your choice
- 1 cup of fruit, your choice
- 1 oz. chopped dark chocolate
- 1 ½ cup milk of your choice (more or less if you want it thinner or thicker)
- 1 tsp real vanilla (extract will work to start)
- Sweeten to taste. Since fruit is already sweet, use ½ banana, or a handful of dates to sweeten further

Blend, blend, blend.

I am open to change!

Tip 1: Add vanilla protein powder or a few tablespoons of collagen! You can also sneak in ground flax, or chia, seeds. Nuts too! This smoothie should never remain the same.

Tip 2: Try to keep out "added" sugar. The point in these recipes is to make food fun, to take control of the food, but to be more intentional and healthier. With a little thought, most food can still taste amazing and be better for you.

Tip 3: Be brave! Add small amounts of things you normally wouldn't eat but want to put into your day: kale, spinach, or other greens. Make the amounts small to start and work your way up slowly.

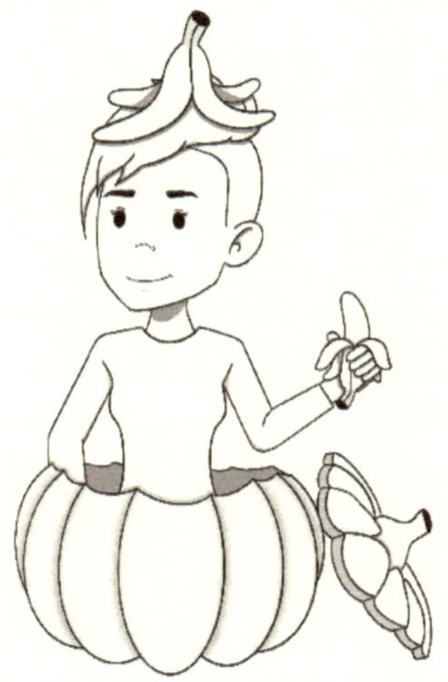

I Am a Scientist

Record your thoughts!

- Do I question things? Do I think of possible scenarios?
- Do I research things so I can make a decision that is better for me?
- If a decision I make doesn't work out, do I give up? Or do I try again?

____

____

____

____

I am a scientist.

I love to question things. That's what scientists do. What if I do this? What if I do that? If I have a question or problem or a tentatively brilliant idea, I will do hours of research to gather information until I'm satisfied.

I learned in my coaching education that when it comes to diet, there is never only one answer. So, I experimented with many different options, took what worked for me, and then kept learning and experimenting. I have fallen in love with this process! And you will too!

One such example of this scientific process was intermittent fasting. My son, Dallas, was doing it. He explained it to me. I knew I needed to learn more. I began reading about it, listening to podcasts about it. I watched Ted Talks and learned about it from countless other authorities.

My son and I discussed fasting more and more frequently. Finally, I knew I had to give it a try. As with everything, it required practice.

I found that even if I didn't change the food I ate and simply did the intermittent fasting eating pattern, I felt so much better. Once I got the pattern down, I combined it with eating better. The two combined provided incredible results such as better sleep, better mood, and more energy—just to name a few. Had I not been willing to question what I was doing, to learn and research, and to practice and experiment with intermittent fasting, I would not have discovered its benefits. I would have missed out on so many wonderful changes to my health and life overall.

Be the scientist of your life. Question, research, learn, and experiment. As you make this recipe, think of yourself as a scientist. Say out loud the phrase:

I am a scientist!

Sound funny? It's okay. Go ahead and laugh, but say it anyway. Say it as you measure and pour each ingredient. Say it as you mix. Say it as you pour the mixture onto the griddle or waffle maker. You are the scientist of your kitchen and of your life. What kind of tasty, cool pancakes can you come up with?

I Am a Scientist – Pancakes Exercise

I paired pancakes with this learning moment because I have made at least 50-60 pancake possibilities in my kitchen—much to my children's chagrin. Confession...at least a handful didn't turn out so well. There is never a pancake made the same in our house. Ask my kids and grandkids. It's an adventurous gamble on every plate of pancakes.

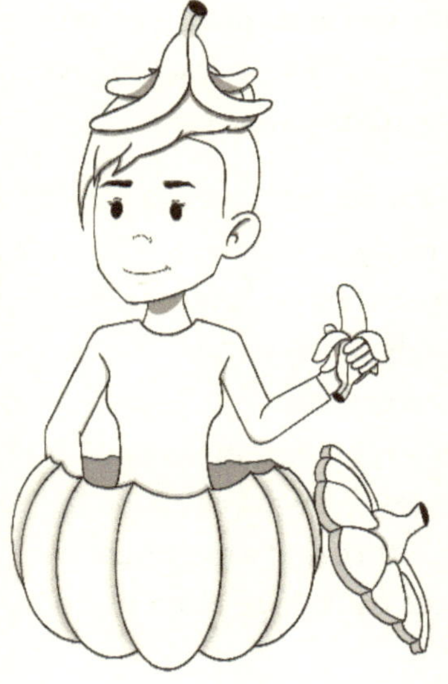

Why? Because I am a scientist!

Variation 1 – Pumpkin Pancakes
Ingredients:

- Pancake mix: choose your own pancake base. There are so many kinds these days that are high protein, paleo, gluten-free, and more. I like to use a gluten-free mix from the store, but you can use a homemade pancake recipe as well.

Here is a homemade pancake mix example:

Flour – 1 ½ cups (all purpose, non-bleached, or one of the whole wheat kinds). Baking powder, 3 ½ tsp. Sea salt, ½ tsp. Milk (of choice), 1 ¼ cups. Egg, 1 large. Vanilla, 1 tsp. Oil or butter, 3 tbsp. (remember, grass-fed butter). Oil spray for pan or griddle (I use an olive oil spray.)

- 6-8 oz can of pumpkin
- 1 scoop collagen, or vanilla protein powder
- 1 tsp real vanilla (extract is okay)
- Almond milk (amount is based on the pancake mix you use)
- ½ tsp cinnamon (or more to taste)
- ½ tsp ginger (or more to taste)
- ¼ tsp cloves
- ¼ tsp nutmeg
- ¼ tsp cumin

I am a scientist!

Create:

1. Follow the directions on your pancake mix, adding in the extra ingredients. Mix well, but do not over mix.
2. Heat an electric griddle to 350 degrees (or a large frying pan on medium-to-medium-high heat). Grease with a little grass-fed butter or cooking spray.
3. Pour ¼ to ½ cup of pancake mix for each pancake. Flip after 1-2 minutes. Adjust flip time as necessary (I am intuition! I am a scientist!).

Part of being a scientist is to smell the aroma, to pay attention to your results and make notes for tweaking the recipe the next time. Don't be afraid to develop your own variation!

Tip 1: The added pumpkin not only flavors the pancakes; it makes them moister. If you want them more cake-like, add more protein or collagen.

Tip 2: Once you've poured the pancake batter onto the griddle, you can sprinkle the pancake with nuts or other toppings as desired.

Tip 3: You can use regular milk in this recipe to replace the almond milk. But I like the extra nutty flavor that the almond milk provides.

Tip 4: Top with grass-fed dairy butter and *real* maple syrup. Trust me, good syrup makes a difference and is a great alternative to cheap sugar syrup. It is a little more costly, but you can use less by melting the butter and pouring them together. Absolutely delightful!

Tip 5: Do not limit yourself! You are the scientist of your life. Brainstorm and create your own crazy, tasty pancakes!

Variation 2 – Banana Pancakes
This recipe is the same as Variation 1 except the banana replaces the pumpkin. Want more cinnamon? Ginger? Other spices? Add more. The spices can be adjusted every time you make these recipes until you get the flavor you want.

- 2-3 small ripe bananas

Create:

The instructions to create are the same as Variation 1.

I am a scientist!

Part of being a scientist is to smell the aroma, to pay attention to your results and make notes for tweaking the recipe the next time. Don't be afraid to develop your own variation!

I Am a Scientist pancake recipe:

____
____
____
____
____
____

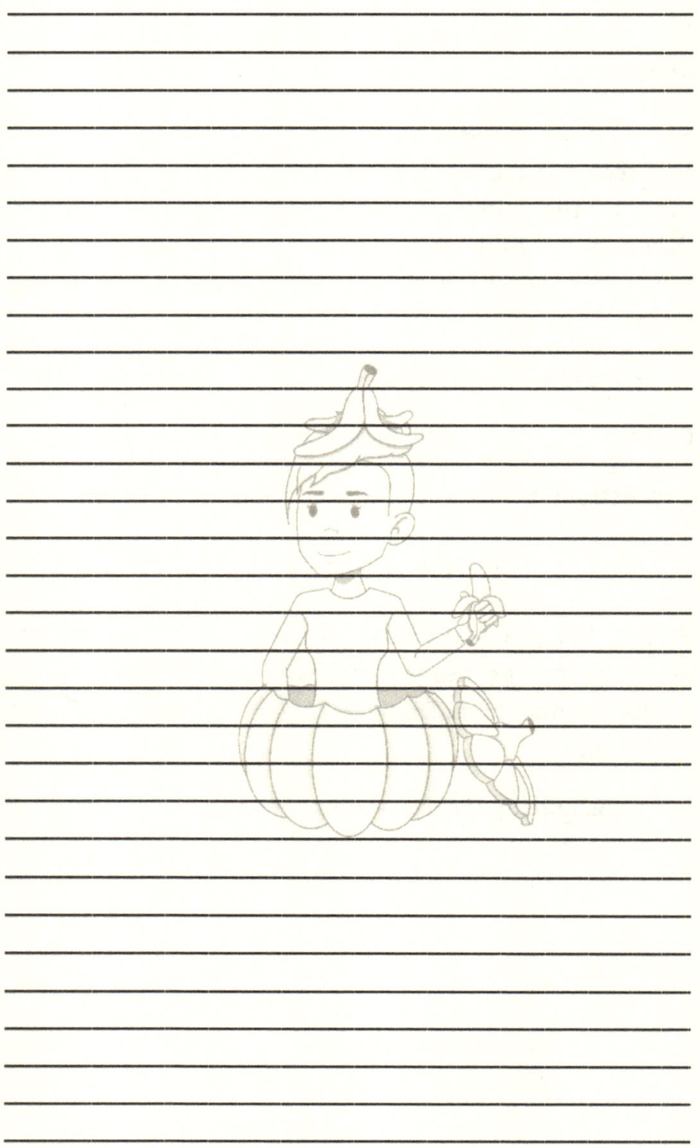

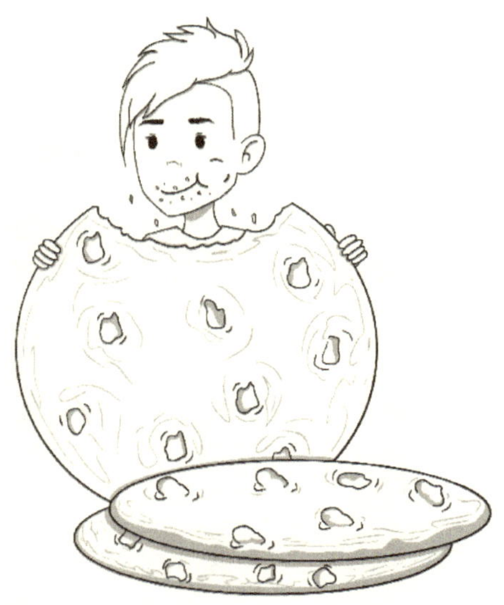

I Am a Relationship Expert

Record your thoughts!

How do I feel about myself? Do I like myself? Do I accept me as I am? Am I willing to change to like myself better? Where do I see myself headed?

____

____

____

____

____

____

____

We are all relationship experts.

One of the most important relationships you will ever have is the relationship with your body.

What you think and feel about yourself is more important than the food you eat. Yes! Let's say that again.

What you think and feel about yourself is more important than the food you eat!

Look in the mirror. Yes, right now. Get up and look in the mirror. I bet you will immediately find at least three-to-five things you wish were different or that you don't like. Maybe even more. That self-talk right there, that is the relationship you have with yourself.

Truth: working on this relationship with your body is a lifelong process. It can be good, then bad, then okay, and then great. It is how it is. But what is important about the relationship you have with your body is that you praise it for all that it does for you. It works 24/7/365 to keep you alive and kicking despite the crazy things you say and do to it. Now, that is amazing!

Now imagine for a moment that every time you look in the mirror you see your nose and you don't like it. You say to yourself, "Ugh! I wish I had a cute nose. Why is it so small? Why is it so crooked?" As soon as you realize what you are saying and doing, change what you are saying to yourself to, "Nose, you may be small and crooked, but you are mine. You helped me smell those amazing pancakes this morning. You helped me smell the rain this afternoon. Without you I would really look funny. I am so thankful I have you. Thank you for all you do for me."

Practice this with *everything* you see that you don't like. You can also give credit to the parts of yourself that you like. "I love my hair. I have amazing legs." Take time every day to be grateful for a body that breathes, smiles, walks, digests your food, allows you to drive a car down the street...you get the idea.

There is no more profound relationship on this planet than the one you have with yourself. How old are you? That is how many years of relationship experience you have. You are a relationship expert!

As you make this recipe, I want you to say out loud the phrase:

I am a relationship expert!

As you make these scrumptious, almond flour, peanut butter cookies, think of the yummy goodness you are about to enjoy. Close your eyes as you take that first bite. Smell the peanut butter and vanilla aroma. Feel the texture in your mouth. Ponder how it melts in your mouth.

Your brain loves to experience satisfaction and euphoria. Imagine if you treated all of your relationships this way. Now that would be a relationship we could all fall in love with. You *are* a relationship expert.

I Am a Relationship Expert – Peanut Butter Cookies Exercise

My advice up front: double or triple the batch. It will be a delight you are going to want to share!

Ingredients:

- ½ cup almond flour
- 1 cup all-natural peanut butter
- 1 egg, large
- 1/3 cup granulated sugar (easily substitute Swerve, monk fruit, Truvia, or coconut sugar)
- ¼ tsp baking soda
- ½ tsp real vanilla (extract will work)

I am a relationship expert!

Process:

- Preheat oven to 375 degrees.
- Combine the peanut butter and egg with the sugar. Mix in vanilla.
- Combine dry ingredients. Mix well. Add to the wet ingredients. Combine but do not overmix.
- Consider refrigerating for 30 minutes to an hour for a stiffer batter. It makes forming balls easier.
- Line a baking sheet/cookie sheet with parchment paper or silicone for best results.
- Roll spoonful of batter into approximately 1-inch ball, roll in granulated sugar, and set on baking sheet 2 inches apart. Slightly flatten balls with a fork. Make crisscross pattern for a traditional appearance.

- Bake for 7-8 minutes, but adjust as needed for your kitchen. Over-baking these cookies makes them very dry. Cool for at least 5 minutes, but preferably 10. Their consistency isn't "finished" until they have cooled. End consistency should be crunchy or slightly chewy.

Tip 1: Enjoy with milk (regular, almond, or coconut)

Tip 2: Share these with someone you love

Tip 3: Eat slowly

Tip 4: Try experimenting with different "nut-butters"

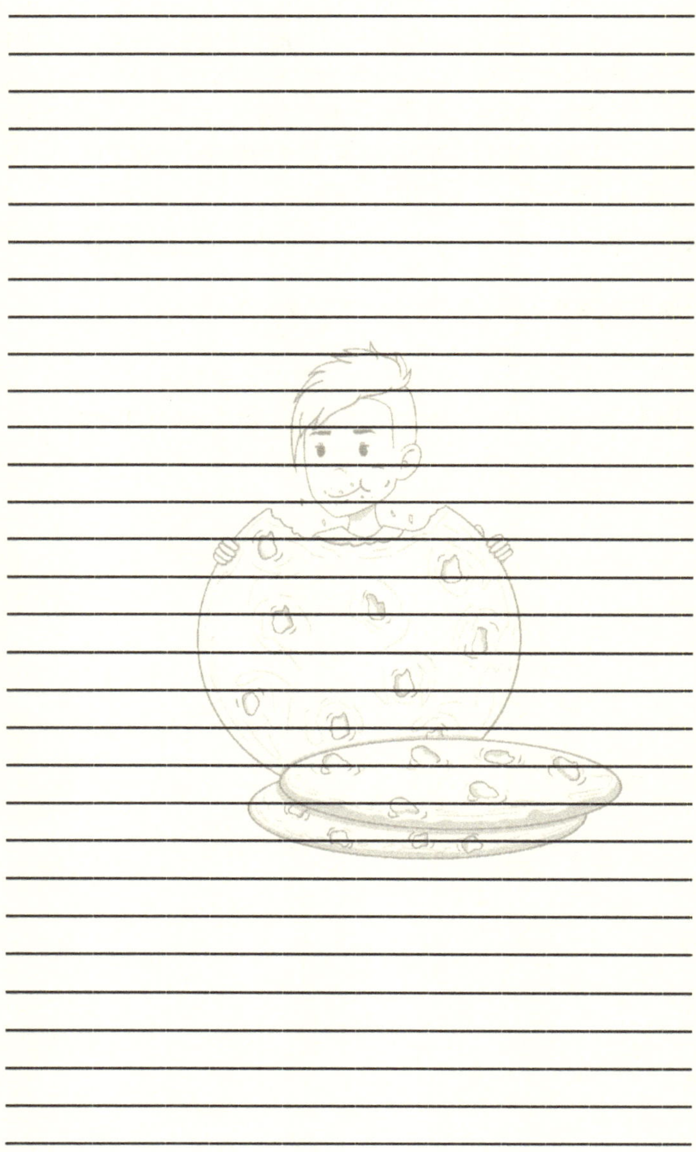

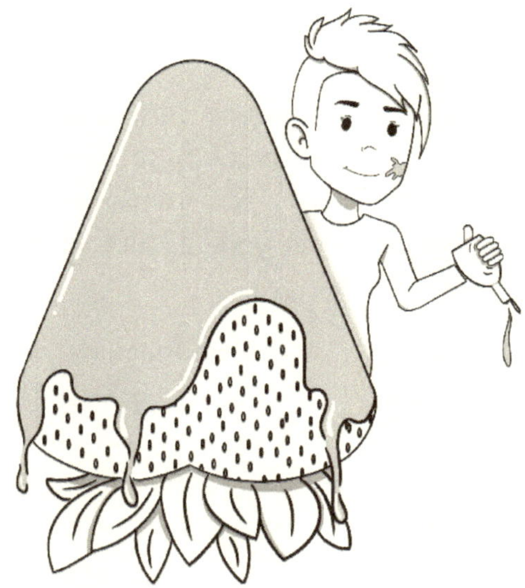

My Intention is the Solution

Record your thoughts!

- What do I want to feel more of?
- How do I want my day to go? How do I want to feel when my day comes to an end?
- What people do I want to love today?
- What things will I check off my list today?
- How do I feel about how I spend my time? What do I want to see? Am I able to be me?

____

____

____

____

____

____

Your intention is the solution to your problem. It is what drives your every decision.

Every decision or action you take around food has a positive intention, whether it is to stop your stomach from growling or to soothe your soul from an argument you had with a loved one. Maybe you had a rough day at work or you are feeling lonely.

So much of what we do is surrounded by food. Your body works the same way. Every craving or desire has a positive intention. You might be short on magnesium today and so that causes a reaction. Your body is trying to communicate. Maybe you are tired and cannot seem to ever find enough energy to do what you need to do, like playing with the kids or get out and walk and enjoy the outdoors.

Your cravings are not the problem. They are what your body and mind see as the best solution you have at the time. Being aware of the deeper meaning behind these cravings and behaviors is the key.

I know I want to live a long and healthy life. I joke all the time about living to be 91 years old. Why 91? I took a quiz about six years ago on livestrong.com. It asked a bunch of questions about eating, lifestyle, stress, etc. The final estimate it gave me was 91. I think at the time I was particularly worried about living long enough to see my children grow into adults. When you are a single parent you worry about what the story will be if you ever leave this life early and what (and who) will happen to your kids.

My intention was to get confirmation that my life would be long. Funny huh. No matter what questions we answer on a website, unfortunately they will not guarantee longevity!

What I got from that experience, though, was far more. I realized I wasn't doing that bad and that I definitely needed to fix some things so I could make that happen. This has silently guided my life in interesting ways. My intention is to grow old and be around to be the matriarch of my family and to love and serve all of those around me. With this intention, my choices are directed in a way that will lead me there. Intention guides my life, from how I spend my time, to what job I work, to who I spend my time with, to what I eat, to how often I exercise, to how I drive my car, and the list goes on.

As you make this delightful treat and take each bite, say out loud:

My intention is my solution!

Then, hum with happiness as your mouth waters with each strawberry and chocolate morsel!

I chose this delightful healthy dessert because I want you to eat each spoonful with intention. Enjoy. Relish. Bask. Let this represent your intention to eat good food – food that's good for you—in the most fun and intentional way. Own each choice, each meal, each path. Believe that your intentions are the best solution you have come up with so far...until you learn and grow again and again. Every intention will be replaced with a new and improved intention.

My Intention is My Solution – Dessert Exercise

Step 1: Choose your yogurt (4-8 oz.)

Dairy-free coconut yogurt or any other choice will work. I suggest vanilla flavor to begin with. It goes amazingly well with chocolate and fruit.

Step 2: Choose your chocolate (1-2 oz.)

I suggest you use a dark chocolate. It's lower in sugar and real cacao is very good for you. However, you get to choose the chocolate that you love and feel is good for you.

Step 3: Choose your fruit (1/2 cup)

You can use one or several fruits. The idea is to make this decadent and full of delight. I suggest raspberries or strawberries. Blueberries work too. However, you could also add mandarin oranges and peaches.

My intention is my solution!

Step 4: Create:

1. Scoop the yogurt into a bowl.
2. Chop the chocolate into small chunks or shave into curls and slivers. A cheese grater works great for this!
3. Sprinkle on your fruit of choice. Mine is strawberry!

Tip 1: It's so important to eat this dessert intentionally. To do that, take small bites. Pay attention to how it tastes from beginning to end. Chew slowly so you can identify and notice each flavor before you swallow. Close your eyes and intentionally enjoy it, being mindful of all the nutrition your body is receiving.

Tip 2: Brainstorm! Now, go and make your own variation!

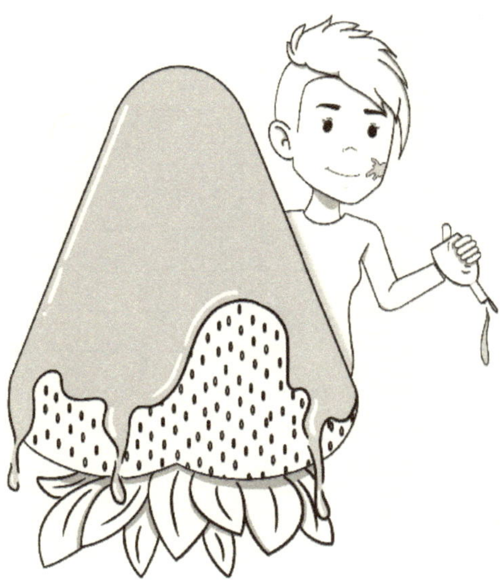

My Intention is the Solution dessert recipe:

____

____

____

____

____

____

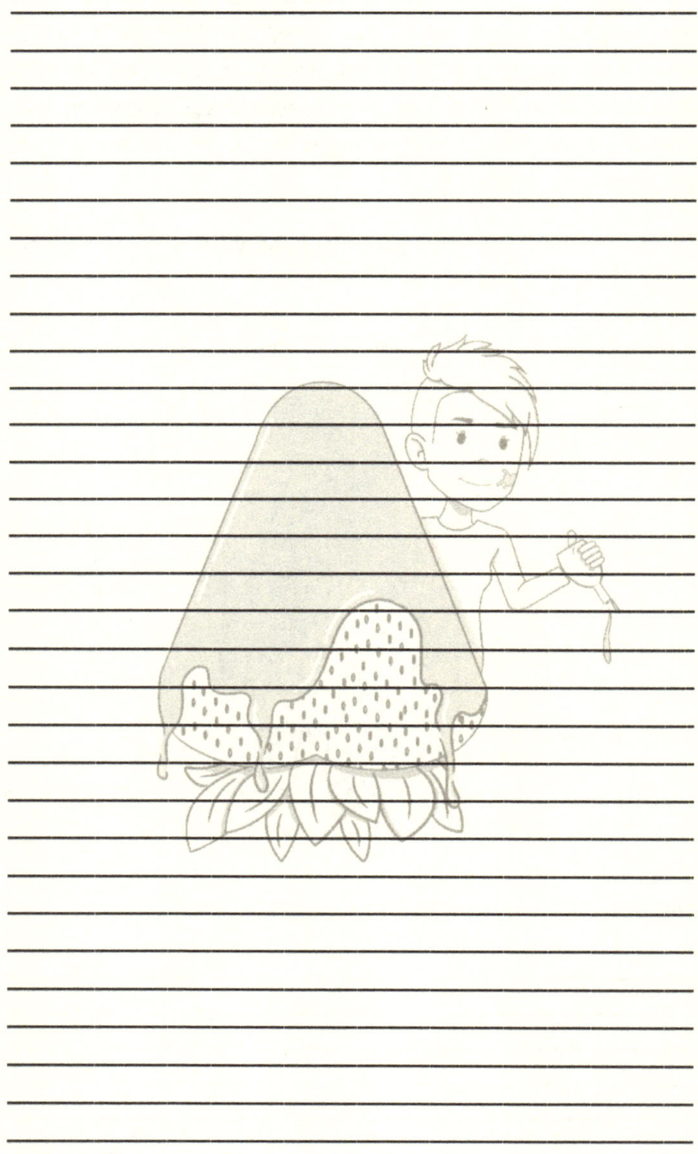

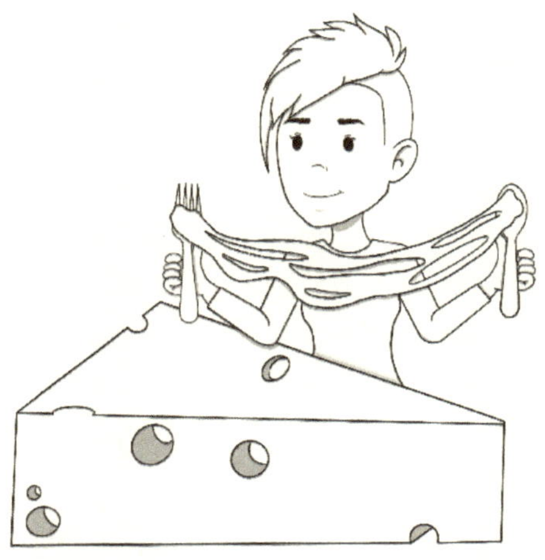

I Feed My Soul

Record your thoughts!

> Do you feel better when you listen to music? Do you find comfort in reading and getting lost in a story? Does the sunshine make you feel alive?

____

____

____

____

____

____

____

I feed my soul. Do you feed your soul?

Our bodies require more than food as nutrition. You can have a seemingly healthy body but not be fulfilled mentally, emotionally, or spiritually. This can be a deep abyss.

I know I have balance in my life when I feel impacted by small things. Just the other day I had a tight feeling in my chest. I was feeling like I couldn't quite get that deep breath. I found myself wondering if I was doing my best at my job and I kept thinking, "Am I ever going to reach my health and fitness goals?" and so on. This went on for the better part of the day.

Suddenly, the noise in the room was so loud I couldn't think. I was overwhelmed and frustrated about things that never usually bother me. It was that moment that practice has taught me that I have overlooked myself and focused on other things and other people. This happens in some way to all of us. Many times, it is unavoidable.

We try not to get to this point, and yet many times we find ourselves there. My training and experience have taught me that this is when I need self-care the most. For me that includes a 6-7 mile walk along the mountain close to my house. Feeling the breeze and sunshine on my face. Pondering the incredible size of the mountain I see. Thanking my creator for such an amazing thing to put my life into perspective and humble me.

Self-care for me is also a podcast by one of my favorite biohackers, or inspiration from an icon like Tony Robbins or Oprah Winfrey as they share experience and insight. Self-care for me is the pleasure I get from making food I know fuels my body and sets me up for success. It smells wonderful, tastes good, and makes my body feel good afterward. Self-care is beautiful music by Mozart, or an exciting throwback of a band I remember from high school. This is how I feel my soul.

As you make this macaroni and cheese recipe, I want you to say out loud the phrase:

I feed my soul!

Pour self-love into this wonderful creation. Find joy in making it yours after tackling the initial recipe. Do some self-care while you take each bite by eating it with someone you love, while watching your favorite movie, or sitting on a sun-warmed porch with your eyes close and letting each bite melt in your mouth.

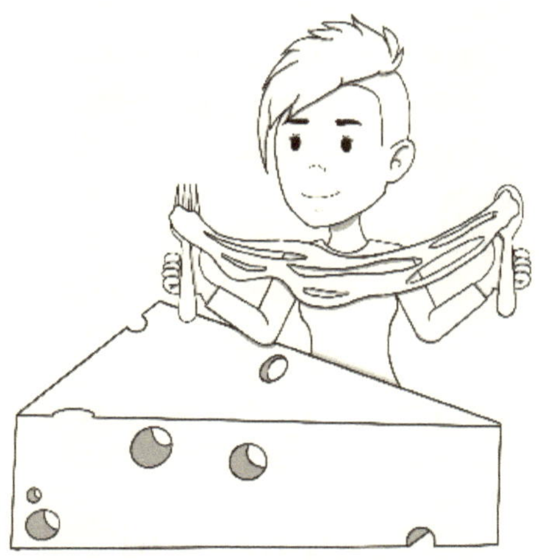

I Feed My Soul – Macaroni and Cheese Exercise
I'm going to suggest a few possible variations on this recipe. But feel free to experiment!

Step 1: Choose your pasta

You can use regular semolina-based pasta, chickpea, vegetable-based, or even legume pasta.

Step 2: Choose your cheese

Cheddar is popular, but you can use parmesan, pepper jack, Colby jack, a shredded store mix (Mexican, pizza, Italian), Havarti, gouda, or do your own combination.

Ingredients:

- 1 box pasta
- 2 cups shredded cheese (do three cups if using real Parmesan-Reggiano)
- 1/8 tsp red cayenne or 1 tsp sriracha
- ½ tsp sea salt (table salt will also work)
- ¼ tsp freshly ground black pepper
- 2 cups heavy cream (do *not* substitute with milk or half-and-half)
- Optional: 1 tsp fresh garlic (or ½ tsp garlic powder)
- Optional: ½ tsp onion powder

One box of pasta usually has 6-8 servings. If you want 3-4 servings, simply halve the recipe.

I feed my soul!

Create:

- Fill a large pot 2/3 full with water. Bring the water to a rolling boil and add 1/8 cup of salt once it is boiling. Add pasta and boil according to package directions.
- In a large sauce pan, bring two cups of cream (with your spices) to a simmer (do not overheat!). Add the shredded cheese and stir consistently until all the cheese is melted. Set aside.
    - If you want to add garlic or onion to your sauce, put 1 tsp of oil in your saucepan (before adding the heavy cream) and sauté the garlic and/or onion powder for about 30 seconds.
    - Remember, the pasta has been cooked in salted water, so don't add more salt to the cheese sauce until tasting it with the pasta.
- When pasta is ready, drain well. Return to pot. Pour melted cheese sauce over the top and stir. Taste. Add more salt if desired as some cheeses are saltier than others. Add more pepper or sriracha to taste.
- Enjoy: This is a great side to a beautiful pile of steamed broccoli or other veggie delight. You can also eat it in a heaping pile, sprinkled with more cheese and additional seasoning. Enjoy with someone you love or wrapped into a blanket watching your favorite movie.

I feed my soul!

Tip 1: It is so important to get the most out of this experience, so take small, intentional bites. Chew slowly so you can fully enjoy all the flavors before you swallow. As you enjoy each bite, be in the moment. Close your eyes and focus on what you created.

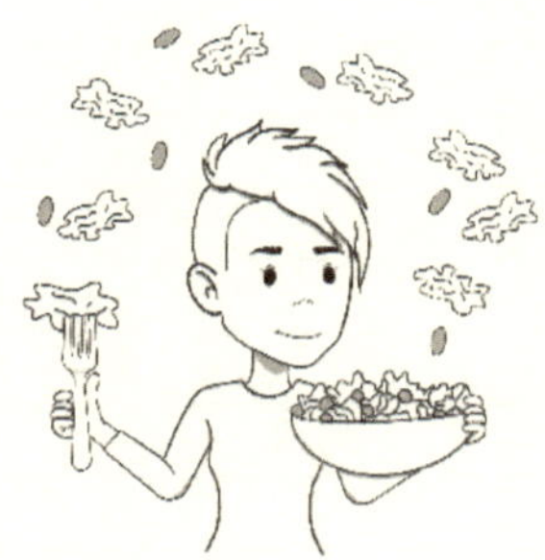

Ingredient Suggestions for Eating Your Best Life

It's always okay to use what you have on hand for the recipes in this book. But, as you embrace "eating your best life," consider acquiring and completely transitioning to healthier, more intentional ingredients. These might include:

Healthier Flour

> If you can eat gluten, do research in your area to find specialized sources that sell less processed flours. For example, where I live, I have access to Abigail's Oven. They sell flour that has been unheated, un-bromated, unbleached, and un-enriched. It's the pure stuff. They also sell amazing Dutch-oven sourdough made with this amazing flour.
>
> While some nice grocery stores are getting better at sourcing less-processed flours, you can usually do much better with a little research.

Healthier Butter

In most grocery stores you can now find butter (and other dairy) from farms that do not use hormones on their livestock. They also grass-feed their livestock so the dairy they do produce is simply healthier and better.

Fresh Fruits and Natural Sugars

Sugar doesn't have to be an enemy. I try to be careful how much cane sugar I eat, but what's more important to me is simply being balanced. Bananas are a great sweetener and can be used in many recipes to sweeten things up without adding extra sugar.

But, when you do need extra sweetness, consider products like Swerve, monk fruit sweeteners (and mixes), erythritol (which is commonly mixed with monk fruit), and good fresh and dried fruits.

Healthier Spices and Seasonings

We all need salt. But, look for salt products that have more minerals. Most sea salt, pink Himalayan salt, and brands like Real Salt are healthier and include many natural minerals that overly processed salt products remove.

Spices are immensely good for you. The key is, the fresher, the better. But, if you don't grow herbs in your garden, the next best option is freeze dried. Compared to regularly dried herbs, freeze dried herbs have more flavor and maintain more of their nutrition and benefits.

Grass-fed Meats

Most of the meat sold in stores today is from animals that are grain fed. This means they were fed only grain combinations over the course of their life in a feedlot. Grass-fed comes from animals that eat more of their actual natural diet and are less medicated for sickness. This makes the animal, and therefore the meat, healthier and safer to eat.

Grass-fed animals are able to produce the right amounts of fat, have healthy babies, and are generally treated more humanely. The need for healthier meat is becoming more widely known in our world. However, this meat can still be a bit more expensive in some areas. So, eat meat sparingly, and when you do eat it, eat healthier meats.

Acknowledgements

It is really important to me that everyone who helped bring this project to completion be recognized for their contribution. We all know that nothing worth doing can be done alone. So, with that in mind, I want to thank Kennedy Smith for the initial idea to put together my random recipes. I want to thank Bethany Tolley for inspiring me to add important concepts together that go with my coaching ideals and also what we are always talking about on our podcast, **The Stuff Life Is Made Of**. I want to thank Alea Saunders for helping me with motivation and moral support. I want to thank Dallas Saunders and family for their input and food inspiration and support as well.